Fruits
and
Vegetables

*One Secret
to a
Healthier Lifestyle*

RON KNESS

Contents

Disclaimer

This publication is for informational purposes only and is not intended as medical advice. Medical advice should always be obtained from a qualified medical professional for any health conditions or symptoms associated with them or before starting any diet.

Every possible effort has been made in preparing and researching this material. We make no warranties with respect to the accuracy, applicability of its contents or any omissions.

Introduction

Your parents told you to eat your vegetables as a child. You were ordered to *"clean your plate"* if you wanted any dessert. As an adult, your doctor, fitness coach and multiple health experts extol the virtues of eating lots of fruits and vegetables, and not so much processed food. However, you can't help but wonder, can natural, minimally processed foods like fruits and vegetables really make much of a difference in your life?

If they are so good for you, how come foods like asparagus and Brussels sprouts don't taste anywhere near as wonderful as cheeseburgers and chocolate? If vegetables and fruits are supposed to be so great for overall health, why are there more pizza shops and fried chicken restaurants than fresh fruit and vegetable stands? Have you ever asked yourself these questions? If so, you have unwittingly fallen prey to modern marketing messages by food manufacturers.

Just because something is prevalent does not mean it makes for the wisest choice.

In this book you will learn how to eat more fruit and vegetables every day. In the very next section, you will learn exactly why naturally nutritious vegetables and fruits are such an important part of a healthy lifestyle and could be one secret to living a longer life.

Why Fruits and Vegetables Are So Important

The way the human body processes food has not changed for thousands of years, however, our predominant food supply has. With the advent of modern agricultural and food processing methods, we have seen a lock-and-step increase in heart disease, cancer and other dangerous and deadly conditions.

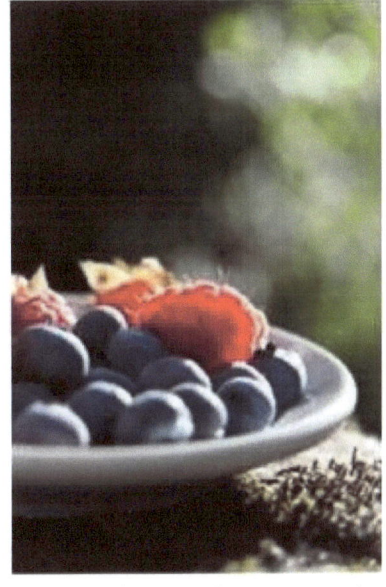

That is because modern-day food is unfortunately highly processed. Salt and refined sugar, monosodium glutamate (MSG) and trans fats, preservatives, steroids and man-made chemicals are intentionally injected into most of the food you eat. This is not done to make you healthier. It is simply done to make the food longer on store shelves, taste better, and to produce as addictive a product as possible (so that you will buy more of it).

Fresh vegetables and fruits (not fried or slathered in unhealthy dressing) have naturally healthy levels of the nutrients, minerals and vitamins your body needs. They do not contain the processed sugar, insanely high levels of salt, steroids, preservatives and other nutritionally bankrupt chemicals found in processed food.

Unfortunately, the fruits and vegetables that human beings once used to eat in abundance are now lacking in most diets. Your body still craves the same nutrition requirements it did when your ancestors were eating healthy foods. However, if you continue to reward your hunger with too much unhealthy processed food, and not enough healthy fruits and vegetables, poor health and debilitating medical conditions will be your reward.

The fact that you are a product of nature, and fruits and vegetables are natural food sources, reveals why they are so important as a part of your healthy diet plan.

You could live the rest of your life in a rather healthy manner without a single teaspoonful of processed, refined sugar. Healthy levels of sodium are found in vegetables and fruits. Processed food delivers incredibly high levels of salt and sugar, and this leads to an extremely elevated risk of contracting heart disease, high blood pressure, obesity, diabetes, cancer, Alzheimer's disease and several other unwelcome and potentially life-shortening health conditions.

Many fruits and vegetables also have a high water content. The human body requires at least 1 gallon of water to be ingested each day to function properly. So simply by eating more fruits and vegetables, you help properly hydrate your body.

Another important aspect of swapping out processed foods for vegetables and fruits has to do with how much you weigh. If you find it hard to lose weight and maintain a slim, trim, sexy figure, your diet is probably to blame.

The last few decades the importance of nutrition as the major health factor has come to light.

As high as 80% of your health and physical fitness is dictated by your diet alone. The other 20% is from exercise.

This means trading a bag of potato chips and a sugary sports drink for a handful of nuts and a glass of water or unsweetened tea during your next snack. Small moves like that begin to impact your health in a positive manner, immediately. Fruits and vegetables are nutrient-rich, low in calories, and they make you feel full longer than unhealthy processed food.

This means you eat less, which lowers your chances of being overweight or obese. That is because vegetables and fruits are high in dietary fiber, but generally low in calories.

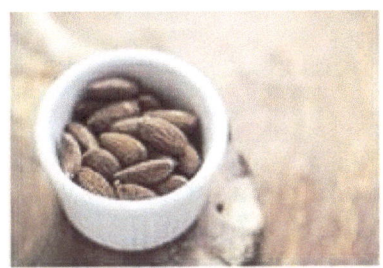

Processed foods have little fiber, and tons of empty calories. Fiber takes a long time for your body to process, which means 1 cup of broccoli will make you feel full faster and longer than 2, 3 or even 4 cups of processed sugar!

Now let's take a look at exactly how much nutritionally healthy natural fruits and vegetables you should be eating.

How Much Fruits and Vegetables Do You Really Need?

Can too much of a good thing be a bad? Concerning eating fruits and vegetables, you really can't (nor will be able to) eat too much. They are so full of fiber, nutrient-dense while being low in calories and carbohydrates, that you fill up quickly and simply can't overeat these wonderfully nutritious foods. That having been said, let's look at what some important health and nutrition organizations have to say about daily fruit and vegetable requirements.

The British Nutrition Foundation

This UK government organization recommends vegetables and fruits should be included at every meal and also at snack time. They first outlined the guidelines for smart eating in 1994. They named these recommendations *"The Eatwell Plate"* in 2007. They recommend that these foods **"make up approximately one third of your total daily food intake."**

Five portions of fruits and vegetables a day is recommended for adults.

The BNF describes a portion as 1 medium-sized piece of fruit. This could be an apple, pear or orange. Small fruits such as plums or apricots require 2 to constitute 1 portion. A portion of vegetables is usually between 3 and 4 heaping tablespoons. You are aiming for about 80 grams (3 ounces) of fruits or vegetables per portion. Fruit or vegetable juices require 150 ml (5 ounces) to make 1 portion.

They point out that choosing from a wide variety of vegetables and fruits is the best way to ensure that you are getting all of the vitamins, nutrients and minerals you need to stay healthy. They recommend eating fruits and vegetables that are in season, as the fresher your food is, the healthier it is.

The BNF offers a free and wonderful resource for educating you on how many fruits and vegetables you should be eating on a daily basis. That free digital download is available at https://www.nutrition.org.uk/attachments/article/720/Fruit%20 and%20vegetables.pdf.

The United States Department of Agriculture

The USDA released their 8th edition of the Dietary Guidelines for Americans in 2015. This includes recommendations from the Department of Health and Human Services in the US. This standard is published every 5 years, and can be found at http://health.gov/dietaryguidelines/.

The USDA recommends consuming *"more of certain foods and nutrients such as fruits, vegetables, whole grains, fat-free and low-fat dairy products, and seafood."* They go on to suggest that their research shows a diet low in added *"sodium (salt), saturated fats, trans fats, cholesterol, added sugars, and refined grains"* provides health benefits.

Specific guidelines used to be called MyPyramid, and are now referred to as the Healthy MyPlate. It is recommended that Americans fill **"half your plate with fruits and vegetables."**

Eight ounces of seafood consumption per week is recommended, as well as never skipping breakfast and increasing **"consumption of plant foods (vegetables, beans and peas, whole grains, nuts and seeds)"**.

The USDA does not speak in terms of serving size, as they state that *"the number of cups of fruits and vegetables your family needs daily depends on caloric needs, which are determined by age, gender and activity level."* However, it should be noted that **1/4 cup was the recommended serving size for one portion** of fruits or vegetables back when the MyPyramid food guide was in effect.

This refers to chopped fruits and vegetables or juice made from those foods. It does not refer to fruit and vegetable drinks which have sugar and other unhealthy ingredients added. Make sure all your meals and snacks are made up of at least 50% fruits and vegetables and you will be on the right track.

Health Canada

Health Canada is the branch of the Canadian government tasked with recommending smart nutrition habits. They publish Canada's Food Guide, which lists the types of food you should be eating, as well as serving sizes, depending on your age and sex.

Adults 19 to 50 years of age should be getting between 7 and 10 servings of vegetables and fruit each day. If you are 51 years or older, 7 daily servings will suffice.

Teens between 14 and 18 are recommended to eat 7 or 8 servings of vegetables and fruit each day, and children should be consuming between 4 and 6 servings daily.

Health Canada refers to 125 ml (1/2 cup) of frozen, canned or fresh vegetable or fruit juice as a single serving. A single medium-sized piece of fruit is recommended as 1 serving, as is 250 ml (1 cup) of salad or leafy raw vegetables.

Other modern countries and communities recommend similar daily requirements of vegetables and fruits as Health Canada, the BNF and the USDA. Be careful though, not all fruits and vegetable servings deliver the same nutritional value, which we will cover in the next section.

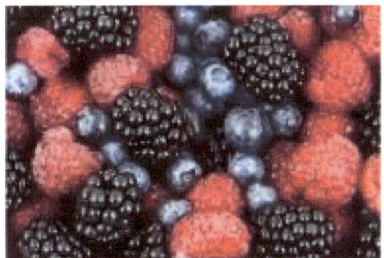

Why Not All Fruits and Vegetables Are Good for You

We mentioned in the last section that juices made with fruits and vegetables containing sugar are not healthy for you. You even have to watch some all natural juice from fruit. For example if you eat an orange, you normally have one orange.

However if you drink a glass of orange juice, you could be getting the juice from up to three oranges. This means you are getting three times the sugar you would otherwise get if you ate just one whole orange.

That brings to light the difference between healthy and unhealthy vegetables and fruits. If you coat your veggies in processed, enriched flour and deep-fry them, you are not creating a nutritious meal.

You should also **choose raw greens and fruits whenever possible.** Simply by heating fruits and vegetables, you remove a small amount of their nutritional value. When you eat food as close to its natural state as possible without tampering with it in any way, you receive the maximum value of the nutrients, minerals and vitamins it has to offer.

When purchasing any type of fruit or vegetable juice or smoothie, check the food label. Any ingredient which ends in -ose reveals the presence of processed sugar. If your smoothie or juice drink lists several hard to pronounce or confusing sounding ingredients, you should probably pass.

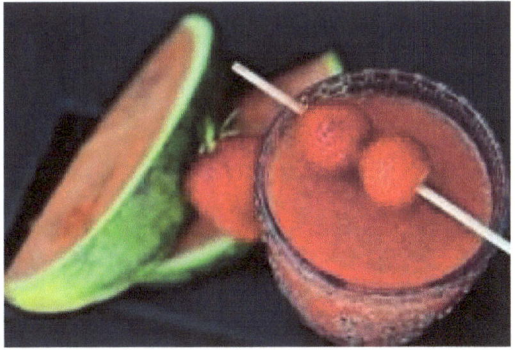

If you don't buy or can't get fresh vegetables, choose frozen over canned. Canned goods often have high levels of sodium. When you order vegetables and fruits away from home, ask your waiter or chef about their quality and preparation. You may find a healthy sounding restaurant dish is actually nothing more than unhealthy processed food.

Juice and vegetable beverages are safe and healthy when they contain nothing but natural ingredients. You should also remember that eating too many fruits and ignoring vegetables can cause you to gain weight. Fruit tastes sweet and delicious because it contains natural sugars. So eating too much fruit could lead to weight gain, though you would have to consume quite a bit to trigger this effect.

Concerning Food Allergies

The most common food allergy is a sensitivity to peanuts. This can range from mildly frustrating to deadly in nature. Concerning fruits and vegetables, some find that they respond negatively to oranges and other citrus fruits. Some people discover that eating apples or celery is impossible.

Every human being is different. Some people simply cannot eat carrots, peaches or cherries without triggering an Oral Allergy Syndrome. You will have to experiment with different fruits and vegetables. Eat them in various combinations and alone. Try eating them raw, steamed and sautéed.

If you find that one particular food causes an allergic reaction, don't worry. There are hundreds of nutritious and delicious fruits and vegetables that can replace the one that doesn't sit right in your stomach.

12 Top Fruits and Veggies to Include in Your Diet

Excellent health is not some secret formula. It is now (and has been for a while) common knowledge that exercise, drinking plenty of water, getting proper rest and eating smart is the formula for health and fitness. However, it wasn't until the last 15 or 20 years that doctors and health professionals have come to realize just how important nutrition is for your overall health.

As much as 80% of your level of fitness, mentally and physically, is determined by what you eat.

This means if you eat a lot of processed foods, full of sugar, trans fats, MSG and other nutritional nightmares, you will be unhealthy. Your risk of contracting cancer, diabetes, heart disease and other possibly deadly conditions will rise proportionately.

But, the opposite is also true (and it is never too late to start).

If you eat mostly fruits and vegetables, you will feel and look stronger, healthier and better. What veggies and fruits should you focus on for optimal health and fitness? Add the following 12 naturally healthy superfoods to your diet starting today, and your health will start to benefit immediately.

1 - Blueberries

These berries (technically a fruit) are known as being some of the most nutritionally complete foods in the world.

You can eat them raw or in baked goods, add them to your cereal or oatmeal, sprinkle them on your salad and use them as the basis for healthy jams and jellies.

Blueberries are constantly referred to as one of the healthiest foods in the world because they contain one of the highest antioxidant densities of all vegetables, fruits and spices. Antioxidants combat free radicals that cause damage to your cellular

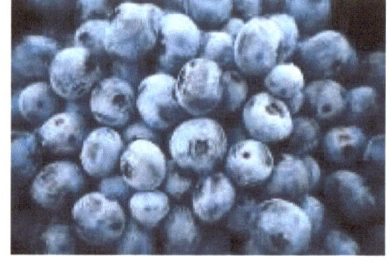

structure and even your DNA. They help regulate a healthy blood sugar level, promote a healthy immune system, deliver heart healthy cardiovascular benefits and improve mental function.

2 - Avocado

This versatile food can be eaten raw, processed, cooked and included in a wide number of recipes. Though often referred to as a vegetable, the avocado is a fruit, technically a berry. Interestingly, bananas and apples release a naturally occurring hormone that causes avocados to ripen quicker when these fruits are near each other.

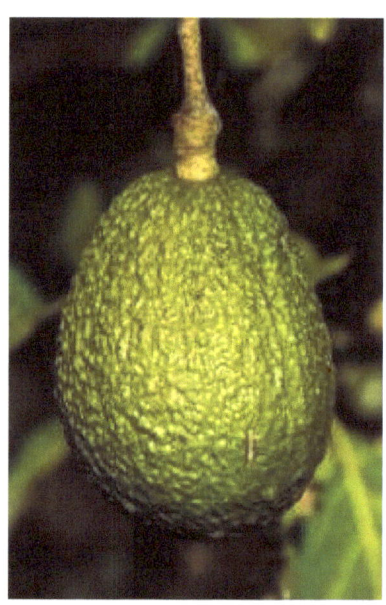

The healthy monounsaturated fats found in avocados boosts heart health, and mashed or puréed avocado can replace unhealthy butter in many recipes. The antioxidants and amino acids in avocado are excellent for treating damaged, dry hair and skin, sunburns and even wrinkles. This fruit is rich in vitamin K, copper, folic acid, dietary fiber, vitamin B6, vitamin C and potassium.

3 - Spinach

Popeye's favorite vegetable is rich in vitamin C. Spinach can be eaten raw, steamed, baked, boiled, broiled and cooked just about any way you can imagine. Spinach is also found in healthy juice recipes, and delivers the most health benefits when consumed raw. It makes a great addition to scrambled eggs!

Incredibly, just 1 cup of spinach provides from 24% to 987% of 13 essential nutrients your body needs. Full of fiber, vitamin K and A, manganese, magnesium, iron, copper, vitamin B2 and B6, spinach delivers multiple health benefits. It offers amazing anti-inflammatory and anticancer properties and promotes a healthy immune system.

4 - Cranberries

Cranberries deliver a sharp, pungent and tangy flavor. They can be used to make jellies and jams, and can be eaten raw, dried or cooked in a multitude of recipes. Cranberries are 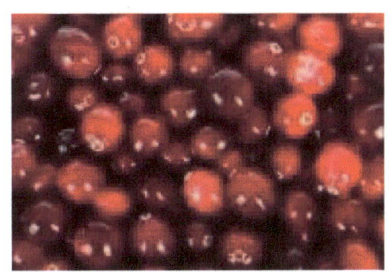 actually grown in bogs and then floated in water to make harvesting easy.

This convenient harvesting method also exposes floating cranberries to high levels of sunlight, which increases the amount of healthy phytonutrients this super-healthy food delivers.

Eat cranberries and you will limit your chance of contracting urinary tract infections (UTIs). Rich in manganese, vitamin C, dietary fiber and vitamin E, cranberries have anti-inflammatory and anticancer properties. They also strengthen your natural defense system and boost cardiovascular and heart health. This is another food rich in antioxidants which protects your cellular structure and DNA.

5 - Kale

Kale is just as easy-going as the other foods on this list. It doesn't care how you decide to eat it, raw or cooked, it still delivers incredible health benefits. This leafy green vegetable has over the last few years become very prevalent in the juicing community. Combined with spinach as a base for a salad, you would be hard-pressed to find a healthier vegetable combo.

Kale is excellent for detoxing your digestive system. It has been linked to lowering your chances of contracting cancer of the prostate, ovaries, breast, bladder and colon. It is rich in dietary fiber, fights chronic inflammation and delivers healthy immunity system-boosting antioxidants. Just 1 cup of cooked kale provides between 20% and 1,180% of all the copper, manganese and vitamins K, A and C that you need on a daily basis.

6 - Banana

Did you know that banana plants can grow as high as 30 feet? A single cluster of these fruits can hold as many as 150 bananas.

With natural sweetness and a creamy but firm flesh, the banana is delivered from nature in a bright yellow jacket. Add slices to your cereal, enjoy a delicious banana raw, or use bananas as the base for spreads, 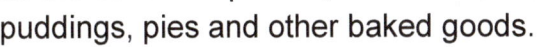 puddings, pies and other baked goods.

One medium banana delivers 25% of your vitamin B6 daily requirements. You also receive between 10% and 16% of biotin, copper, fiber, potassium, vitamin C and manganese. Those nutrients and minerals deliver cardiovascular health, and can help regulate a healthy blood pressure. Bananas also help your digestive system work properly, and are known to boost athletic performance.

7 - Prunes and Plums

Plums arrive naturally in a wonderful rainbow of colors. They can be sweet or tangy, and are at their most nutritious and delicious when eaten raw. The annual plum season runs from May through October. Plums belong to the Prunus genus along with peaches and almonds, as well as their cousin the prune. (Prunes are actually European plums which have been dried.)

Vitamin C and K, copper, fiber and potassium deliver the health rewards of plums and prunes. The level of phenols in these fruits leads to outstanding antioxidant protection. Your brain cells and cell membranes are composed of high levels of fat. The antioxidants in prunes and plums protect against oxygen-based damage to those fats, and these fruits also normalize blood sugar levels, keep you "regular", lower high cholesterol levels and can promote weight loss.

8 - Cucumbers

Cucumis Sativus is the scientific name for this wonder-

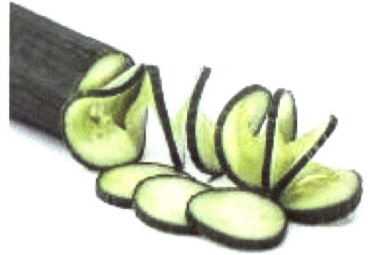

vegetable. While the classic cucumber is recognized as long, green, and cylindrical in appearance, there are actually dozens of varieties that come in all shapes, sizes, textures and colors. The type of cucumber you are probably most familiar with is categorized as a slicing cucumber. This vegetable is in the same family as squashes and melons.

Lariciresinol, pinoresinol and secoisolariciresinol are 3 polyphenol lignans found in cucumbers. These health boosters reduce your risk of contracting heart and cardiovascular diseases and multiple types of cancer. Cucumbers also fight inflammation and free radicals, prop up your immune system strength, and deliver vitamin K, potassium, copper, manganese, vitamin C, vitamin B1 and at least half a dozen other essential nutrients.

9 - Romaine Lettuce

A single leaf of romaine lettuce delivers varying degrees of texture and flavor. Romaine lettuce is as versatile as kale and spinach, and as healthy as well. Most of the romaine lettuce sold in the United States comes from California and is delivered through a year-long harvest.

Use 2 cups of romaine lettuce as a healthy base for a salad and your body benefits from 20 essential nutrients, minerals and vitamins.

Folate (also known as vitamin B9) and vitamins K and A are found in high concentrations in romaine lettuce. This low-calorie, nutrient-rich vegetable actually slows down the aging process of your heart. Romaine lettuce protects your blood vessels, can help lower high blood pressure, and reduces your risk for contracting heart disease.

10 - Apple

If you think the 2,500 varieties of apples grown in the United States is an impressive figure, consider this. There are more than 7,500 apple varieties grown throughout the world. Commercially, only about 100 different types of apples are marketed. Those include the popular Golden Delicious, Fuji, Macintosh, Red Delicious and Granny Smith varieties.

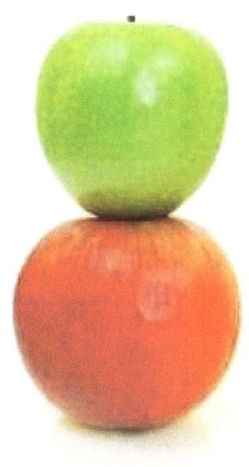

You have probably heard the old saying that *"an apple a day keeps the doctor away"*. That comes from the fact that apples deliver phenolic acids, anthocyanins, phytonutrients, vitamin C and dietary fiber that combine to offer several health advantages.

This is another of nature's antioxidant providers. Add apples to your diet and you enjoy a lower risk of contracting asthma, lung cancer and cardiovascular problems. Healthy blood sugar level regulation and anticancer benefits are also delivered.

11 - Carrots

These crunchy, orange veggies are more than just Bugs Bunny's favorite food. Carrots are easy to pack and carry, high in nutrition and low in calories, and are generally available throughout the year. In your local area, carrots are most probably harvested in the summer and fall, and this is when they are full of healthy nutrients, minerals and vitamins, as well as the most flavorful.

The beta carotene in carrots promotes excellent eyesight, especially night vision. Beta-carotene also delivers cancer-fighting and cell-protecting properties. Just 1 cup of carrots (raw) gives you a full 17 different essential nutrients, minerals and vitamins. These include vitamin A, vitamin K, fiber, potassium, vitamin C, B6, B3, B1, B2, E and biotin. Carrots promotes a healthy heart and cardiovascular system as well.

12 - Celery

Celery does not receive the respect it deserves as a healthy part of a nutritious diet. Because of its high water content and lack of a strong flavor, this crunchy, low-calorie vegetable is often overlooked as a healthy food. However, the under-appreciated celery delivers a laundry list of impressive health benefits.

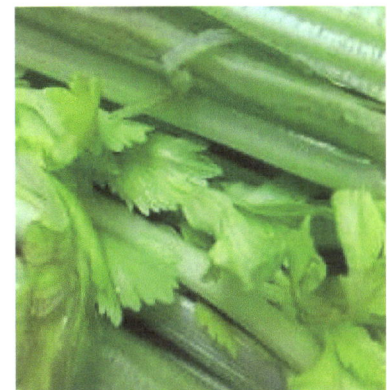

Antioxidants such as vitamin C (along with blood vessel and organ protecting flavonoids) help boost a healthy immune system.

Celery offers powerful anti-inflammatory properties as well. It helps regulate a healthy digestive tract, and provides you with 15 essential nutrients.

Your blood vessel walls, heart, entire cardiovascular system, digestive tract and risk of contracting cancer are all positively affected when you eat this super-food. Celery is also one of just a few vegetables that doesn't lose a significant amount of healthy nutrients, vitamins and minerals when it is boiled or cooked.

7 Ways to Eat More Fruits and Veggies Every Day

You may be thinking, *"How do I get more fruits and vegetables into my daily diet plan?"* The following 7 tips will make sure that you are eating plenty of healthy natural foods, and fewer processed food items.

1 - Start Juicing

The juicing revolution is in full effect around the world. Purchase an inexpensive juicing machine, and you quickly and easily turn several servings of fruits and vegetables into a delicious and healthy beverage. If you would like more information on juicing, get my book Fight Cancer with Juicing. It is available at: https://www.createspace.com/6155567.

2 - Add to Your Favorite Foods

Diced broccoli and onions can complement your favorite whole-grain pasta. Add fruits and vegetables to a couple of eggs and make a healthy omelet. Start incorporating vegetables and fruits into other foods that you already enjoy.

3 - Keep a Bowl of Fresh Fruit in Your Kitchen

Having a bowl of fresh fruit on your dining room table or kitchen counter is a good way to promote healthy eating.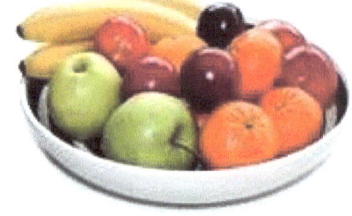

4 - Drink 100% Fruit or Vegetable Juice

Make sure your juice is 100% natural. Steer clear of juices that say "contains vegetables" or "made with real fruit". This could be a sign that only a portion of the juice is healthy. Limit yourself to 8 ounces per day to avoid adding too much natural sugar to your diet.

5 - Play the Replacement Game

As mentioned in Tip #3, you are going to eat what is available when you are hungry. Replace processed foods and unhealthy beverages with fruits and vegetables in your refrigerator and freezer.

6 - Prepare Bulk Lots

Why not cook and prepare a week's worth of vegetables and fruits on the weekend? You can do this in just an hour or two, and package by serving size so you and your family can benefit from quick and healthy meals with little preparation and cleanup.

7 - Make Your Own Soups

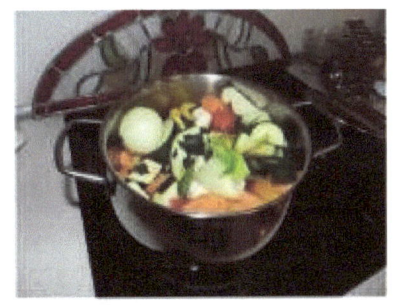

Store-bought canned soup is usually ridiculously high in sodium. It can also contain other unhealthy ingredients. Make your own soup with your favorite vegetables in a crock pot, and freeze individual serving sizes.

6 Food preparation Tips to Save Time and to Eat More Fresh Food

It is possible to save time while eating more fresh food. Enjoying a healthy diet does not have to eat up big chunks of your time. The following 6 food preparation tips help you eat more fruits and vegetables and enjoy the health benefits those foods deliver, while saving you time in the process.

1 – Keep Frozen Vegetables on Hand

Bulk size and single serving portions of frozen vegetables are available in most supermarkets and grocery stores. This requires little preparation and cleanup, allowing you to eat healthy without a big time investment.

2 – Make a Plan

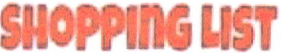

When you plan your meals a week at a time, you control just how much fruits and vegetables you eat. Set aside 1 day each week to write out a meal plan, and then use that as a basis for your shopping list.

3 – Purchase Several Single Serving Containers

Choose 4-ounce to 8-ounce re-sealable glass containers. Plastic can contain unhealthy BPA's, and glass allows you to tell with a glance exactly what food is contained inside.

Purchase as many single serving containers as you need to make the next tip possible.

4 – Cook Once, Eat All Week

This is virtually the same advice as Tip #6 from a previous section. You cook one time for the entire week. You then portion out serving sizes and store in your refrigerator and freezer for quick and easy access, with little cleanup.

5 – Buy in Bulk

When you buy vegetables and fruits in bulk you can save a lot of money. This also saves valuable time, as you spend less time shopping and running back and forth from your home to the grocery store.

6 – Get the Whole Family Involved

Not only does more hands reduce the workload for everyone involved, but they then have a vested interest in the food when served.

Final Thoughts

Incorporating more healthy fruits and vegetables into your diet is not that hard to do if you use the food lists and tips in this book. If you family is used to eating less than healthy, don't convert them cold turkey. Instead gradually phase in a healthy fruit and/or vegetable and phase out an unhealthy processed food. Most likely they will not even notice.

Next week do the same thing and before long, you'll have them eating healthy and they will thank-you for it. That might be stretching it too far, but at least you'll know they are eating healthy while at your table.

And if they learn to eat healthy at your table, their kids will learn those healthy habits also, so the effect you have now is not only for the current generation, but for many to follow.

Just like a cycle of bad eating habits can be carried down through generations, so can healthy eating. Make it happen and watch your health improve.

Other Health and Fitness Books by This Author

If you would like to read more about Senior Health and Fitness, here is a list of the titles, CreateSpace links and descriptions:

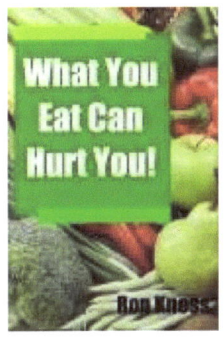

What You Eat Can Hurt You

https://www.createspace.com/4963196

Do you know that certain foods increase your risk for inflammation, disease and illness? It's true! And certain foods can help cure and heal you if you do get sick. Knowing which foods to eat and which ones to avoid empowers you to manage your own health.

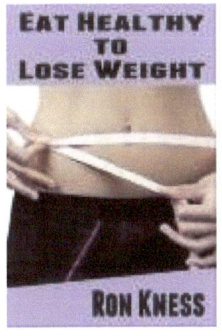

Eat Healthy to Lose Weight

https://www.createspace.com/4962939

As you read through our book, we show you which foods you should and should not be eating to reach your weight loss goal, along with discussing how to maintain your weight loss and stay within a few pounds of your goal weight. Banish the weight you keep gaining back each time by learning how to live a healthy lifestyle.

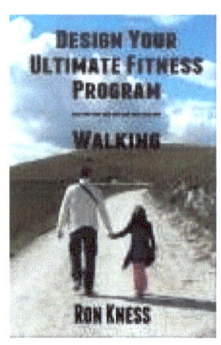

Design Your Ultimate Fitness Program - Walking

https://www.createspace.com/5252272

In my book Design Your Ultimate Fitness Program – Walking, we discuss the considerations that need to be made when designing a custom walking program, along with:

• Equipment needed
• Wearable technology you can use to track your walking
• And how to make walking more challenging

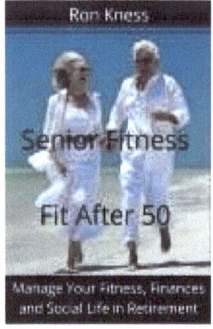

Senior Fitness – Fit After 50: Learn How to Manage Your Fitness, Finances and Social Life in Retirement

https://www.createspace.com/5474751

Inside you will discover answers to your most pressing questions:
• What do I need to know about downsizing my home?
• What are the best tips for staying healthy as you approach your 50's?
• When should I start planning for retirement?
• I am worried about being lonely once I retire, do others feel the same?
• Is it worthwhile to carry two homes during retirement?
And more…

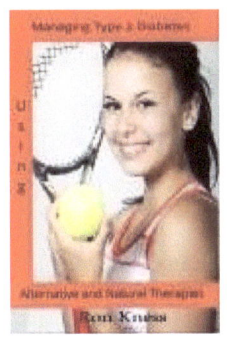

Managing Type 2 Diabetes Using Alternative And Natural Therapies

https://www.createspace.com/5401244

While Type 2 diabetes can be managed medically, there are many alternative natural and holistic methods of therapy and treatment that can further enhance quality of life and minimize the effects of this disease. In this book, I discuss 12 different types, including yoga, reflexology and acupuncture to name just three.

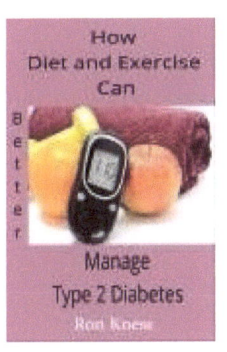

How Diet and Exercise Can Better Manage Type 2 Diabetes

https://www.createspace.com/5404845

Of the different types of diabetes, only Type 2 can be reversed. In my book How Diet and Exercise Can Better Manage Type 2 Diabetes, we reveal the three things you can do to best manage your disease, including:
• Diet
• Exercise
• Weight management

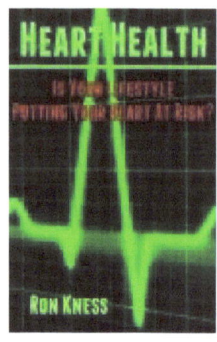

Heart Health: Is Your Lifestyle Putting Your Heart at Risk?

https://www.createspace.com/5464020

In my ebook Is Your Lifestyle Putting Your Heart At Risk? we discuss the six greatest risks to your heart and the lifestyle changes you can make to mitigate them.

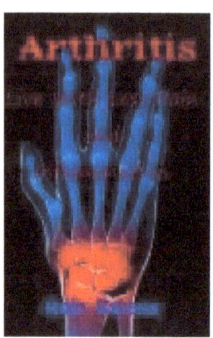

Arthritis – Live Wth Less Pain and Inflammation: Tips and Techniques You Can Use to Lessen the Pain and Inflammation

https://www.createspace.com/5457441

Discover Simple Tips & Information That Will Help Reduce The Painful Symptoms Of Arthritis!

You learn things like:
• Simple and effective information that will help you manage the pain and inflammation that comes along with arthritis, so that you can live an active, full life without debilitating pain.
• The different types of arthritis, their symptoms and how to alleviate their painful side effects.
• The pros and cons of over-the-counter arthritis medications, plus simple tips that will help you know how to choose the right supplements.
• Free, yet effective ways to get relief from arthritis pain and inflammation, so you don't have to suffer anymore.

the effects arthritis can have significant impact on your physical and mental well-being, but this books shows you how to overcome its painful symptoms and live life relatively pain free.

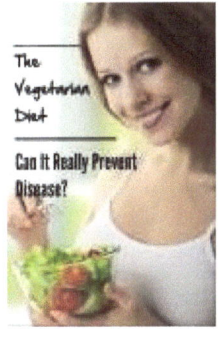

The Vegetarian Diet – Can It Really Prevent Disease?

https://www.createspace.com/5519874

Is a vegetarian diet right for you? Multiple studies have shown over and over that a vegetarian diet goes along way in preventing certain chronic diseases, such as:

• Heart Disease
• Cancer
• Diverticulitis
• Type 2 Diabetes
• Hypertension
• Obesity
• Kidney Failure

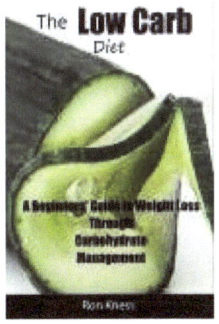

The Low Carb Diet: A Beginner's Guide to Weight Loss Through Carbohydrate Management

https://www.createspace.com/5416348

In my book "The Low-Carb Diet – A Beginners' Guide to Weight Loss Through Carbohydrate Management", I reveal a successful method of losing weight based in part on the amount and type of carbohydrates you consume.

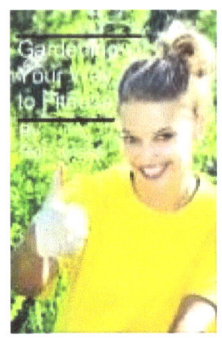

Gardening Your Way to Fitness: The Fun Way to Get Fit and Provide Beauty and Healthful Bounty for Your Family

https://www.createspace.com/5459564

The gym is a great place to stay fit during the colder seasons, but once the temperature turns warmer you want to spend more time outside. Plus, you'll have the benefit of fresh wholesome produce to enjoy by growing vegetables in your backyard garden.

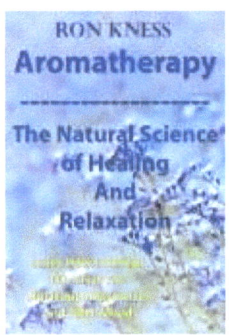

Aromatherapy - The Science of Healing and Relaxation: Learn How Essential Oils Elicit The Relaxation Response And Alter Mood

https://www.createspace.com/5714434

In my book Aromatherapy – The Science of Healing and Relaxation, we reveal the natural holistics methods you can use to heal the body from certain medical issues and to relive stress through relaxation. In particular we talk about:
• Aromatherapy - what it is and how it works
• Essential Oils – how the effects of certain aromas differs from others
• Recipes – how to make your own essential oil combinations

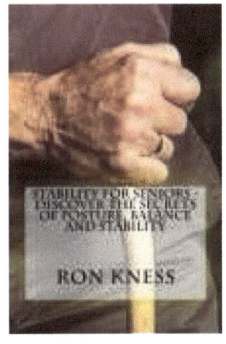

Stability for Seniors: Discover the Secrets of Posture, Balance and Stability

https://www.createspace.com/6096479

Many people sacrifice their health in pursuit of their career. They are so busy making a living that they neglect to make a life. The excuse that they do not have time to exercise is tossed about so frequently that they end up letting their health and fitness slide.

If you are not regularly active, you will have muscular atrophy over time. Your flexibility will decrease. Your core strength will diminish. As time progresses, you will be less limber and more rigid.

This is exactly how people age poorly. It's a process that has snowballed over time.

Only with regular exercise and a healthy diet can you have a body that is fit and has the ability to almost reverse aging.

If you have neglected your health for years and life seems to be a chore now because you can't get around without assistance, do not feel dejected.

You can remedy the situation. You can restore the strength, balance and stamina that you have lost. It is never too late to become what you might have been.

This guide will show you exactly what you need to do to restore your balance, strengthen your core and give you the ability to live life to its fullest. Read how …

About the Author

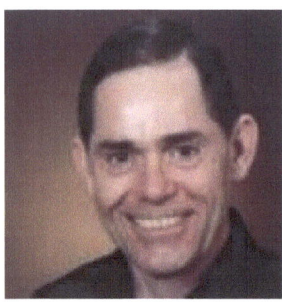

I grew up in Central Minnesota, where my parents owned and operated a fishing resort. Once out of high school I tried a couple of semesters of college, only to quit halfway through the Spring term; I decided at that time that college wasn't for me.

Then I decided to follow my father's previous occupation as an auto mechanic. I graduated from a two-year of vocational training course and worked as a mechanic. While in vocational training, I decided to join the National Guard where I eventually ended up working full-time for 32 years.

So how does all of this relate to writing? In one of my leadership schools, the instructor, who was an English teacher at a juvenile detention center, presented writing to me in a whole new way - a way that started to develop my interest in working with words.

Fast forward about 40 years and I now have over 50 books listed on Amazon for Kindle and CreateSpace.

Besides my own writing, I also ghostwrite ebooks, reports, articles, blogs and do Kindle conversions for my clients on a variety of topics.

Today my wife and I live in Gold Canyon, AZ, where you'll find me happily sitting in my office typing away on my laptop as I work on my next book or ghostwriting project . . . that is if we are not traveling on a cruise ship - our new-found mode of travel.

www.ingramcontent.com/pod-product-compliance
Lightning Source LLC
Chambersburg PA
CBHW050855290526

45792CB00002B/608